Also by Dr. Stenbeck

Available from the usual on-line source

Books
Healing Yourself -- The Holistic Approach
[An introduction to Holistic Self-healing.]

Heal Yourself Right Now!
[The Seven Priority Organ Levels for
effective Nutritional/Holistic Treatment of
all organs.]

The 22 Unique Body Types
(for Health and Weight Loss)

Q & A to Identify Your Body Type (Booklet)
[Individual Type booklets are also available

Booklets
(Step-by-step instructions on healing yourself)

> *#1 Start Healing with Positive Thinking*
> *#2 Mastering Positive Feelings for Health!*
> *#3 Spiritual Balance and Your Healing*

The Carboferic Body Type

Representing one of the 22 Body Types first described by Victor Rocine around 1900

The Bill Murray, Roseanne Celebrity Body Type

For Kaye,
there at the beginning with Doc Severn,
and for Liberty,
continuing the holistic healing journey…

Disclaimer

About the Author

Educated in New Zealand and in the U.S.A., Dr. Stenbeck attained B.Sc. (NZ), M.S., and D.C. degrees. His holistic healing methods have been profiled in magazines (Esquire, McLean's, Playgirl, the Atlanta Constitution), and on TV in the USA and in Canada. He was the main contributor to the Warner Book, _The Eye/Body Connection_ by Jessica Maxwell that focused on the holistic healing relationships between the iris structure and organ genetics.

In the 1970-80's he was elected Fellow, Royal Society of Health, London; Fellow, American Association of Chemists; Member, American Association of Clinical Chemists; and Affiliate, Royal Society of Medicine, London. He studied naturopathy and Body Types with Dr. Bernard Jensen and Dr. Clifford Severn, and has practiced in medical partnerships where patients received the joint benefits of medical and holistic healing.

He is a member of Self-Realization Fellowship. To receive advice on any health issue from a holistic viewpoint, or to receive help with your body type, see his web site: *DrStenbeck.net*

―――――

Contents

* * *

The Carboferic Body Type and Food Guide   1

---

* * *

The 22 Body Types:
Celebrity Examples

This Booklet contains the Carboferic type. See
The 22 Unique Body Types for all type
descriptions.]

Thin Types

Atrophic	*Woody Allen / Audrey Hepburn* *Stan Laurel / Calista Flockheart*
Exesthesic	*Cher / Sarah Jessica Parker* *(Female type only)*
Marasmic	*President Obama / Princess Diana* *James Stewart / Kate Blanchard*
Neurogenic	*J.K. Simmons / Joan Rivers* *Jon Cryer / Marin Hinle*
Pathoferic	*(No celebrity males)* *Blythe Danner / Gwyneth Paltrow*
Sillevitic	*David Bowie / Shirley MacLaine* *Rod Stewart / Carol Channing*

Muscle Types

Calciferic	*Michael Jordan / Angelica Huston*
	Abraham Lincoln / Grace Jones
Carbogenic	*George Clooney / Lady Gaga*
	Pres. G. Bush, Jr. / Meg Ryan
Desmogenic	*Marlon Brando / Loni Anderson*
	Daniel Craig / Tina Turner
Eldic	*Ross Perot / Hillary Clinton*
	Peter Falk / Sigourney Weaver
Myogenic	*Pres. Bill Clinton / Sharon Stone*
	Pres. John Kennedy / Julia Roberts
Medeic	*Gary Oldman / Madonna*
	John Hurt / Marlene Deitrich
Nervimotive	*Frank Sinatra / Elizabeth Taylor*
	Mark Wahlberg / Natalie Wood
Nitropheric	*Ben Affleck / Ava Gardner*
	Kirk Douglas / Kate Winslet
Pallinomic	*Pres. Donald Trump /*
	Attorney General Janet Reno
	Bill O'Reilly (Fox) / Jane Russell

Fat Types

Barotic	*Robin Williams / 'Mrs. Doubtfire'* *Elton John / William Conrad*
Carboferic	*Bill Murray / Roseanne* *Billy Gardell / Melissa McCarthy*
Hydripheric	*John Goodman / Shelly Winters* *Wayne Knight / Jennifer Holliday*
Isogenic	*Einstein / Oprah Winfrey* *Phillip S .Hoffman / Queen Victoria*
Lipopheric	*Rush Limbaugh / Rosie O'Donnell* *Chris Christie / Camryn Manheim*
Oxypheric	*Winston Churchill / Orsen Welles* *Ella Fitzgerald / Gerry Spence*
Pargenic	*Burt Reynolds / Katey Segal* *Ron Perlman / Kirstey Alley*

<u>*Succinct Quote on Human Types*</u>

From Victor Rocine, who first described discrete body types around 1900.

"A type is an order of people that differentiates and distinguishes itself by a general and similar form, brain-formation, chemistry, structure, build, immunity, tendencies, predisposition, resemblance, skin-pigment, and type characteristics based on observation and analogy.

"Or, in other words, people of a given type are similar physically and like-minded as if they were brothers and sisters—that is what type means.

"Everything in nature is made according to plan. Man only discovers that plan and gives it a name. The zoologist has not made the animals—he has only described the plan adopted by the wonderful Creator, and named the classes, sub-classes, etc.

"How important type research will be to humanity, time alone will make known."

———

Prologue

The esteemed scientist J. J. Berzelius, discoverer of several chemical elements, inspired Victor Rocine to research body types and to investigate the correlation between types and their diseases. Around 1890-1910, Rocine privately published his original findings on the mineral basis of different body types, and this present book exists because of his brilliant insights.

For many years, I studied with Dr. Clifford Severn who had been a personal student of Victor Rocine on body types, naturopathy, herbology, iris analysis, diet, and nutritional healing methods. He had a successful career as a lecturer and healer, and was one of those rare athletes with complete muscle control over his body. I saw him under a spotlight at 85 years of age, contracting and rippling every individual muscle in his perfectly developed body. Field-Marshal Jan Smuts, the WWII South African Prime Minister, devoted a full chapter of his autobiography to how Severn's healing methods had saved his life. In the 1950's, *Life* magazine did a four-page spread on Severn and his family. Fame he had.

Another Rocine student I studied with, Dr. Bernard Jensen wrote of Rocine's body type research and nutritional methods in his privately published, *The Chemistry of Man*.

This book is deeply rooted in Rocine's original work, and with that of Herbert Shelton, M.D., Ph.D. (at Harvard University in the 1930's). I integrated their research with newer dietary and nervous system data along with celebrity examples of each type, hopefully, making this material easier to digest and more entertaining for the reader.

Gayelord Hauser, another Rocine student I knew, was a celebrated health book author. He wrote a popular book on Rocine's types in the 1940's, *Types and Temperaments;* reputedly, he also introduced yogurt to the western world.

This book exists because of Rocine's creative brilliance and original discoveries in natural healing.

▶ *Rocine: "The soul creates the body type."*

Rocine taught that the soul chooses a body type and brain to live in, thus presenting different experiences and life lessons to master. Why were *you* born the way you are?

That is something to think about, especially if it is true! What would your soul purpose be to live in a particular body type. I provide some thoughts on this issue in each type description and try to assess from my experience with your type the particular lessons of life presented therein.

Rocine was as brilliant in his way as an Abraham Lincoln, Michael Jordan, Michael Phelps, Tony Robbins, or a Daniel Day Lewis—all *calciferic* types—rare, leaders, innovative, brilliant, and highly intelligent in their different fields of endeavor.

Celebrity examples exist for most types, not a duplicate of you, but someone who has your essence in their body-mind individuality. Knowing your type allows you to become a better you!

The celebrity examples provide further help in identifying your body type.

▶ *Rocine's classic findings are the backbone of this book. Integrated with Sheldon's research and with other dietary and food issues including mental, emotional, and spiritual attributes,*

Many people take nutritional supplements and try different diets without a doctor's advice. If this is your choice, use common sense, listen to body responses, and discontinue any allergic reactions to foods or nutritional substances.

———

The Carboferic Body Type

"You may also have a physical or psychological feature not representative of your type such as height, weight, appearance, talent, weakness, strength, etc., due to biochemical errors, environmental influences, racial or cultural differences, and congenital or genetic issues. Nevertheless, the type identification of the average person is usually clear."

—Victor Rocine

Carboferic Type
Celebrity Examples

If you think this is your type, be sure to look at **on-line photographs** *of these examples. Look for general similarities to yourself. Note that sub-types cause the differences in appearance between members of the same type.*

———

ACTING

Richard Dryfuss   Paul Giamatti
John Goodman   William Brimley
Danny Devito   Bill Murray
Dan Ackroid   Jason Alexander
Paul Giamatti   John Arnold

TV

Merv Griffin   Dom Deloise
Alfred Hitchcock
Leo McKern (BBC: "Rampole")

Roseanne Barr
Billy Gardell & Melissa McCarthy ("Mike
   and Mollie")

ARTS/OTHER

David Viscott, MD (psychiatrist)
Henry Kissenger

SPORTS

Babe Ruth   Pete Rose
Fernando Valenzuela

(Many examples are found in baseball, football etc., where muscle-brain coordination is required.)

Read the types, and if still confused you may choose to use the personal request for type identification from my web site: *DrStenbeck.net*

———

Carboferic Type Questionnaire

These questions describe the generic type, and not specifically you! If any question ever applied to you, then choose the True answer!

For Question 1 only:

A = True	*B = Maybe*	*C = Untrue*
15 points	*7 points*	*1 point*

1. Physically identify with celebrity example ____

Then...

A = True	*B = Maybe*	*C = Untrue*
5 points	*3 points*	*1 point*

---

2. Height is close to:
   Males: 5'4—6'6   Females: 5'0—5'9 ____
3. Usual weight is close to:
   Males: 160—450+ Females: 150—330+____
4. Overweight, moderate or obese;
   short or tall ____
5. Muscles moderate to high strength ____
6. May be sensitive, nervous, high-strung ____
7. Forehead lower (high in some) ____
8. Hair lovely, luxuriant ____
9. Nose often smaller than average,
   may have pinched nostrils ____

10. Fleshy face, subtle cheekbones, no cheek indentations _____
11. Teeth white, weak, attractive _____
12. Mouth is narrow _____
13. Skin lovely, whitish when young; ages gracefully _____
14. Some have "beady" eyes _____
15. Have many anxieties and concerns _____
16. Very sociable with anyone _____
17. Loving, sympathetic, congenial _____
18. Good sense of humor: many comics _____
19. Hard-working, serious work ethic _____
20. Gourmet tastes (many enter food professions) _____
21. Able to talk and entertain for hours with humor _____
22. Sensual instincts highly developed _____
23. Usually absent or sparse chest hair; medium to very large bust _____
24. Claim can hold liquor; some cannot _____
25. Voice soft, kind, sympathetic _____
26. Dislike hard physical work _____
27. Lead and rule by gentle persuasion _____
28. Lips full, affectionate, attractive, and may be 'puckered' in center _____
29. Often have pale skin _____
30. High sex drive, some desire sex daily _____
31. Inclined to metaphysics, unorthodox religions _____
32. Love sweets, cookies, ice cream, etc. _____
33. Generally unsuited for military or police (too lenient) _____

34. Musical whether playing, singing, writing_____
35. High level of jealousy _____
36. Tend to be lazy and procrastinating _____
37. Polite and respectful (but sometimes
    not to mates and loved ones) _____
38. Submissive, may be co-dependent _____
39. Many comics, healers, scientists,
    professionals _____
40. Females easily seduced, males good
    at it (and know it) _____
41. May hold grudges for a long time _____
42. May be moody if don't get own way _____
43. Born procrastinators _____
44. Not good in an emergency _____
45. Low blood sugar vulnerability
    (particularly females) _____
46. History of stomach problems _____
47. Alcohol, cigarette, drug, sex
    addictions are relatively common _____
48. Naturally assertive, appear passive _____
49. Often have high blood fats and
    related diseases, diabetes _____
50. Nervous, tense (but not neurotic) _____
51. History of cardio-vascular weakness _____
52. Love those who do much for them _____
53. Outgoing and friendly _____
54. Play and relax hard! _____
55. Slow thinking, but may be brilliant
    and intellectual _____
56. Fleshy hips and abdomen; large
    stomach is common _____

57. Heavy upper arms with thinner wrists, small hands and feet, delicate fingers   _____
58. Short distance from eyes to mouth   _____
59. Crave money, riches, independence   _____
60. Not a strong or forceful personality   _____
61. May act inappropriately at times   _____
62. May appear abrupt at first meeting   _____

▶ *The type questionnaire pinpoints the major features of that type: if the celebrity examples are unhelpful, you may be an unusual variant (in which case ignore the celebrity issue and give yourself 7 points on Question 1).*

Scoring

For question #1:

    A response: give 15 points   = _____
    B response: give 7 points   = _____
    C response: give 1 points   = _____

For questions #2—62:

    A response: give 5 points   = _____
    B response: give 3 points   = _____
    C response: give 1 point   = _____

    Total of the above points   = _____

Interpretation

139—275: PROBABLY Carboferic type
70—138: POSSIBLY Carboferic type
  <70: NOT Carboferic type

The Carboferic Type

Rocine: "Carboferic means starch and carbohydrate gathering." You utilize more food __carbon__ than other types, making you large, strong, and intelligent. You are attractive, honest, self-activating, humorous, assertive, with very high self-confidence.

———

Y ou have above-average intelligence, high intellectual capacity, strength and brain power, with fat deposition apparent by age 4 or 5. Depending on your sub-type, by late teens the fat deposition is well underway and you may already be fat and potentially obese.

▶ *Rocine: "Your health is sabotaged by waste-acid toxicity from excessive starch and carbohydrate intake."*

You are attractive, relax intensely, work hard, have excellent social skills, display an honest work ethic, and are sensitive and nervous. Bosses appreciate your honesty, and you achieve success as a self-activating individual. You are rarely willing to do the required college work on your own time to learn higher skills for greater success. Some of you settle for too little in life, and expect others to take care of you.

A small percentage of the males are quite short as in Danny de Vito.

––––––

Physical Similarity to Other Types

The fleshy *nitropheric* type (Beau Bridges) looks somewhat similar, but is less fatty and more reclusive.

The *lipopheric* type (Jackie Gleason, Ricki Lake) is also large and fleshy.

The *oxypheric* type (Winston Churchill, Ella Fitzgerald) is outgoing, with a larger head, and potential brilliance.

The *hydripheric* type (President Yeltskin, Shelly Winters) is usually large with water-laden tissues.

––––––

Average Height and Weight

Males: 5'4-6'6   160-450+ pounds
Females: 5'0-5'9   150-330+ pounds

You already know something about this type from their public persona and appearance, whether from seeing them yourself or from the celebrity examples. Blend such insights with the type descriptions and the types of your family and friends to discern their presence in your midst!

––––––

Carboferic Type Description

The type description represents how you appear in everyday society. You may have a sub-type that alters parts of this description.

Think of the celebrity examples as you read the descriptions. You are a fat type. Some of you maintain a medium-fleshy body into adulthood, but you know the fat vulnerability is there. You live in a genetically-ordained fat body: you can lose weight, but it is difficult as most of you do not have the necessary discipline to achieve it. You love eating!

▶*You often have high intelligence and a highly developed sense of humor; the males, particularly, may entertain people for hours with jokes and stories.*

Head — Your head is circular or square-circular (on frontal view); the forehead is low, rectangular, and medium-sized.

Hair — Hair growth is plentiful, lovely, and luxuriant when young, but later you may show a balding tendency starting in the back-head. Fair and brown hair shades are more common in females, with dark brown and black hair usual in males.

Eyes — Eye colors are usually blue, light brown or hazel; the eyes have a sincere and honest expression.

Ears — Your normal-sized ears are set closely to the head.

▶ *There is a relatively short distance between the eyes and the mouth (unlike the isogenic).*

Nose — The nose is usually smaller than normal, often having pinched nostrils.

Face — A fleshy face with subtle small cheekbones and without cheek indentations is common. Usually, the *carboferic* face is not wide like the *lipopheric*, but it may be with a *desmogenic* sub-type.

▶ *Rocine: "If the lower face becomes puffed out it is usually an unfavorable health sign."*

Mouth, Lips and Voice — Your lips are full, affectionate, attractive, and the mouth may be compact, or of normal size and shape. The voice is usually soft, low-pitched, sympathetic, concerned, interested, and kind.

Teeth — The teeth are average-sized, white and attractive, but not strong.

Skin — Your skin tends to be lovely and white-tinted when young, and it ages very gracefully without wrinkle formation.

Neck — You have a thick, muscular, strong, and fatty neck.

Muscles — Your muscles are medium-sized or larger, and of moderate to great strength. You are competitive weightlifters, boxers and professional sports people, etc., and may be the strongest Olympians.

Chest — The males may have a bare chest, or have sparse hair; occasionally a hairy chest is found due to a *carbogenic, nervimotive or pargenic* sub-type. A large bust is usual.

Back and Shoulders — You are heavy, fleshy and strong in the back.

Hips and Abdomen — Typically, you show a heavy, strong, large hips and abdomen.

Arms and Legs — The extremities are fleshy and harmonious.

Joints — Strong bones, joints and tendons are common.

———

Carboferic Personality Traits

If you are this Fat type many, but not all, of the following characteristics are present (you may have overcome or moderated the negatives, but recognize that you may once had several of them).

You may have any of the following traits:

- Dislike upsetting others
- You respect mental superiors
- The mind is slow but efficient
- Have a love of nature and music
- Dislike fumes, smoke, noisy or crude people
- Are honest workers with a serious work ethic
- Crave beef and flesh: difficult to be vegetarians
- Are fearful, nervous and edgy, but not neurotic
- Alcohol, cigarette, drug addictions are common
- Usually not caught exercising; most dislike exercise
- Generally a very high sex drive: may desire sex daily
- You have a highly developed sense of h-umor: many comedians

- Attitude is one of 'cockiness', friendliness, high self-confidence
- Desire food regularly (or become moody from low blood sugar)
- Crave sweets, sugars, cookies, ice cream, etc., that make you sick
- Are assertive or aggressive, but may appear passive due to laziness
- Have gourmet tastes and tendencies (often enter food professions)
- May be inclined to metaphysics, conspiracy theories, hidden meanings, supernatural phenomena
- Are loving, sympathetic, congenial, friendly, and sociable (some males appear brusque at first meeting)
- Are usually diplomatic, polite and respectful towards others (but may not be towards mates, loved ones)

▶ *Generally, you do not have a strong forceful personality. You lead and rule by peace, gentle persuasion, and quiet talk: prior Secretary of State Henry Kissinger being an excellent example.*

―――

Potential Challenges

You may have evolved from or not had these general challenges, so don't dwell on them.

- Tend to be jealous
- Are born procrastinators, some timid
- Easily discouraged, emotionally hurt
- May do incorrect things in an emergency
- Will-power weak, may be lazy and submissive
- Females are obedient and may be co-dependent
- Some inclined to whining, complaining, worrying
- Inclined to be disapproving of something well done
- Tend to be grouchy and moody (from low blood sugar)
- May lack self-control around sex, drugs, alcohol (and deny this)
- Rocine: "You may give up too easily and feel that all is lost; or feel victimized by life."
- [A psychologist friend, out of frustration while treating a large *carboferic* man, said he was like "a beached whale." They both laughed.]

▶ *If you relate to any of these challenges, doing something to overcome them serves your evolution.*

―――

Carboferic Stress Management

You have strong *mental* and *emotional* stress prevention giving you a good ability not to internalize stress into your body. You confront people and issues, and honestly express yourself. *[If needing help managing these stresses, see my prior books.]*

———

Love

Although highly affectionate and passionate lovers, you may not be very intimate in your day-to-day communion with loved ones. The males are very good at seduction (and know it)! The younger females are vulnerable to seduction, your sexual engines being often highly charged.

▶ *Rocine: "Your love is dependent: you love those who love and worship you."*

———

Talents and Vocations

Abilities — *Food industries, arts, decorating, fabrics, marketing, negotiating, finance, computers, buying, selling, science, medicine*

Many of you enter the food and restaurant businesses. I have known or observed you as chefs, actors, artists, office workers, business, medical workers, middle management, and in advertising persons. You are highly intelligent, and work best in a structured environment where your duties are clearly set out. Entrepreneurs are rare in your type.

Inabilities — *High level executives, military, war*

You are found in middle management positions, and work by providing service to others; you are not born for hard work or physical labor, but can do it if required.

———

Carboferic Health Problems

▶ *Your blood profiles often show evidence of abnormal fat metabolism associated with high cholesterol or triglycerides.*

When sick you commonly experience health problems or diseases in any of the following organs and tissues:

Cardio-Vascular System — This system is weak and vulnerable to disease.

Diabetes or Hypoglycemia — Diabetes and low blood sugar are common (fatigue, depression, sugar cravings, etc.); you are easily carbohydrate poisoned; to be healthy you should avoid simple sugars and carbohydrates.

Stomach Problems — You internalize thinking stress into your stomach and intestines causing ulcers and intestinal diseases.

———

Acid/Alkaline Factor

[See Chapter 3 for details on this subject, along with the common symptoms found with people of different nervous system dominance.]

For your health and healing, your nervous system genetics require a specific ratio of acid to alkaline foods. You are born with **intermediate** dominance (between *para-sympathetic* and *sympathetic*), and need *balanced* acid and alkaline-ash food intake. (Ash refers to the minerals left in your body after metabolizing foods.) You may indulge in both food classes. Construct this approximate ratio of food selections:

> *50% Fruits, salads, vegetables*
> *50% Proteins, carbohydrates*

If you stray from this ratio, it is healthier for you to eat about 70% fruits, salads, vegetables rather than more protein.

▶ *Approximate your food ratios. On any particular day, it does not matter if one meal is mostly alkaline and another mostly acid—just try to balance it out for the day! If you make a mistake, try again tomorrow. It is a subjective call that you make, and what is done over time that makes the difference to your health.*

———

The Carboferic Spiritual Factor

Skip this paragraph if uninterested in a philosophical perspective on your type!

If as souls, we choose the brain and body type to spend a lifetime in it could be to learn certain spiritual lessons related to perfecting ourselves, and our humanity, in God's eyes. What lessons does the type bring you? Only you can really decide what those lessons are. You know your weaknesses, faults, and behaviors towards others. You know things about yourself that Victor Rocine could never get from his research subjects when he first wrote about types. So search your mind for the answers.

Each discrete type has challenges of life lessons, spiritual goals, etc., and some of yours may be:

Faith — Your faith is rational and dependent on what you can see and touch.

Fat — You live in a genetically ordained fat body for your own lessons of life, whatever they are. Weight loss is possible, but not easy.

Low Will-Power — Your self-confidence is high, but you need hypnosis or other techniques to amplify your will-power.

Low Self-Control — Alcohol and drugs are the main problem in some of you: emotional therapy helps.

Laziness and Procrastination — Many of you often live by "do nothing today that can be done tomorrow."

Egocentric — Your ego needs considerable stroking: humility please! Some of you think that "the world owes you". It doesn't. You know how intelligent you are: allow us inferiors to express our knowledge and wisdom!

———

A Carboferic Story...

James, age 43, 5'10, 280 pounds, had weight problems from around age 12. His general health was good, except for headaches, nervousness, indigestion, and puffiness under his eyes.

Dietary evaluation showed excessive intake of carbon foods: carbohydrates, starches, grains, breads, animal proteins, sweet fruits, simple sugars, and fats—which he needed to minimize. His diet also showed calcium and magnesium deficiencies, and he needed daily: kelp, Swiss cheese, turnip greens, almonds, brewer's yeast, parsley, corn tortillas, dandelion greens, wheat, and cashews.

James also did stress management work and began losing weight almost immediately, and week by week the headaches, eye puffiness, nervousness, and indigestion completely resolved.

———

Carboferic Mineral Foods

Apply this mineral data to the diet following the Fat type descriptions.

Excessive Foods:

- *Sodium (salted, junk)*
- *Carbon (simple carbohydrates)*
- *Nitrogen (beef, red meat)*

Deficient Foods:

- *Calcium (important)*
- *Potassium (unsalted, non-junk)*
- *Magnesium*
- *Trace Minerals*
- *Sodium (unsalted, junk)*
- *Nitrogen (non-beef, vegetable)*

These deficient nutrients are common deficiencies in your type, and predispose you to ill-health. ill, be sure to use these lists with your <u>daily</u> food intake. <u>If</u> not ill, eat from the food lists 3-4 days weekly for health maintenance.
All food lists are in descending order of concentration and value to you; choose servings of foods in the upper half of each list first!
One serving is ½ cup.

Carboferic Excessive Foods –

Sodium from salted junk foods is excessive in your tissues. To preserve your health and weight control you should avoid junk foods and fulfill your sodium needs from the food list (without using the salt shaker).

Carbon is excessive in your type, so minimize it. Excessive in all people who become fat or obese, it is found in every cell of the body as the basis of life.

Nitrogen from red meat is excessive in your diet (if eaten more than 1-2 times monthly), and is a major cause of your acidity and illnesses.

———

Deficient Foods -

In illness or disease, it is important to correct these deficiencies.

Calcium is often deficient in your type and you thrive on dairy foods. It is highly concentrated in bones, joints, muscles, nerves, heart, teeth, and gums; if you have an illness or disease in any of these tissues, eating dairy, calcium foods and supplements may be a significant healing factor.

Potassium is deficient in your type. It is a dominant element in your tissues and is concentrated in and vital to the health of your muscles, heart, brain and all cells. If ill or diseased, potassium foods and supplements are probably a significant healing factor.

Magnesium is deficient in your type and particularly important for your heart and digestive function.

Trace minerals are often deficient in your type due to emotional stress or poor digestion and absorption.

Sodium from unsalted foods (not junk foods) is deficient in your tissues (see above note).

Nitrogen from poultry, fish and eggs should be taken 3-4 days weekly, with vegetarian proteins like legumes (peas, beans), seeds, nuts and pasta on the other days.

* * *

Minimize
Excessive Foods

Sodium (salted, junk): *0-1 servings/week*

Salt, all fast foods, packaged foods, canned and frozen foods, preserved meats (cured, smoked, canned), sauces (soy, barbecue, catsup, etc.), chips (potato, corn, etc.), dill pickles, sauerkraut, bouillon cubes, peanut butter, salted nuts, crackers, canned or packaged soups, processed cheeses, commercial salad dressings, meat tenderizers.

Note: If you must eat anything on the above list, keep it down to 1/2 cup weekly!

Carbon: *0-2 servings/week*

Simple carbohydrates, starches, grains, breads, sweet fruits, white sugar foods, fats

Nitrogen (animal): *0-2 times/month*

Beef, red meats

Eat
Deficient Foods

Potassium: *1-2 servings/day*
Dulse, kelp, blackstrap molasses, brewer's yeast, rice, sunflower seeds, parsley, un-hulled sesame seeds, peanuts, dates, pecans, yams, beet greens, Swiss chard, parsnips, halibut, Chinese chestnuts, spinach, rye, buckwheat, collard leaves, artichokes, millet, mushrooms, salmon, potato and skins, fennel, broccoli.

Calcium, Magnesium: *1-2 servings/day*
Kelp, Swiss and cheddar cheese, turnip greens, brewer's yeast, parsley, dandelion greens, cashews, blackstrap molasses, buckwheat, Brazil nuts, dulse, filberts, peanuts, watercress, millet, pecan, walnuts, rye, tofu, beet greens, buttermilk, sunflower seeds, yogurt, milk.
Also drink milk: 2-3 glasses/day
(Low-fat, non-fat milk, bone broths and soups are healing foods for you.)

Trace Minerals: *1-2 servings/day*
Kelp, goat's cheese and milk, raw garlic, sprouts, rhubarb, beet greens, peach, alfalfa, ginger, rice, oats, pineapples, dry split peas, blackstrap molasses, seeds, nuts, brown rice.

<u>Eat</u>
Deficient Foods

Sodium (non-junk): *1-2 servings/day*

Scallops, lobster, kelp, scallops, gizzard, butter-milk, celery and juice, lentils, almonds, cheese (Roquefort, cottage), Swiss chard, beets and greens, eggs, cod, salt water fish, spinach, lamb, turkey, pistachio, okra, spinach, sesame seeds, watercress, whole milk, turnips, carrots, yogurt, strawberry, oatmeal, lamb, chicken.

Nitrogen (non-red meats):

Legumes (peas, beans), seeds, nuts and pasta
— as desired
Eggs, poultry, fish — 3-5 times weekly

Note: Eat any other healthy foods you desire, but be sure to include the type food suggestions in your daily choices. One serving is ½ cup.

Note -

The above recommendations are for the generic type. Additionally, you may need from a holistic healer, or nutritionist, something more specific for your individuality.

Carboferic Nutritional Supplements

[Take all supplements with food.]

- **Multi-Vitamins** — *2 capsules/day*

- **Calcium with Magnesium** —
  600 mg/twice daily (with about 200 mg. magnesium)

- **Herbs** —
  Brain detox – Valerian Root or Gotu Kola
  Organ detox – Saw Palmetto or Milk Thistle
  (Take one capsule, twice daily for one month; then one, three times weekly.)

- **Lecithin** —
  Take about 1,300 mg/three times weekly

- **Evening Primrose or Flaxseed Oil** — *1 soft-gel/day with food*

- **Other** —
  Chlorophyll, blue-green algae, green magma, spirulina, alfalfa, or other source.
  (Take as directed: take one, three times weekly.)

Important Carboferic Health Concerns

Outdoor exercise and breathing fresh air is essential for your health and weight-loss, but many of you are couch potatoes!

Your nervous system genetics require the *Fat* type Food Guide for health, and any carnivorous cravings are normal and healthy for you. After age 50, you only need 3-4 flesh days weekly.

CARBOFERIC FOOD GUIDE

Aim for -

50% Proteins, complex carbohydrates
50% Fruits, salads, vegetables
and
50% Raw foods
50% Cooked foods

Lose the salt shaker!
Milk and dairy foods benefit your health.
Take the recommended supplements.

Carboferic Weight Loss

Your body absorbs excessive fat from an early age, and you have great difficulty in losing it. Follow the diet and you will make good progress. Give yourself permission to exercise! It is essential for your fat burning.

- *Stop* eating junk sodium and carbon foods.
- *Protein* drink daily, about 25-30 grams.
- *Eat* your body type deficient mineral foods daily.
- *Follow* your *Carboferic* guide (as above).
- *Exercise*: your body type requires only light daily exercise (like yoga, walking, roller-skating, etc.).
- *Simple sugars*: stop all white table sugar and high-fructose corn syrup and drinks containing these sugars.
- *Instead of diet pills,* you need glucomanin supplements that swell and take up space in the stomach thus preventing over-eating.
- *If hypoglycemic* (low blood sugar, fatigue, depression, etc.), which stops fat loss and usually initiates more fat production, it is vital to deal with this problem: take *pantothenic acid,* 500 mg/twice daily with food (see my earlier books).
- *Calories:* As with any dietary approach, calories in, must be *less than* calories out! Most markets sell a calorie booklet; make notes of your daily intake, and in most instances keep it under about 1500-1800 calories/day.

―――

Fat Types
General Food Guide

(An Intermediate Guide between Carnivores and Vegetarians)

Important Note

―――――

The Food Guide addresses the <u>Acid-Alkaline</u> aspect of your food intake, along with the <u>Type Mineral</u> factor presented throughout this book. It does <u>not</u> necessarily address calories or other dietary factors that may be pertinent to your personal health needs whether medical or appropriate for some other dietary need. So use your common sense and just include the factors described here with whatever healthy dietary choices you usually make.

For other nutrient information, consult with nutritional books or with holistic nutritional doctors. In this regard, I particularly recommend the advice of Andrew Weil, M.D.

―――――

Fat Types
General Food Guide

This chapter presents an <u>Intermediate</u> Food Guide, balanced between the Muscle types (carnivores) and the Thin types (vegetarians). Superimpose the individual type mineral and other information from your type chapter into this Food Guide (which is not for the pargenic type.)

––––––

Meat/Flesh Intake

Generally, animal protein is acceptable and needed in your diet: red meat should be limited to once weekly or less, while lamb and fish or poultry are excellent in moderation. If this diet is similar to what you are already eating, but you have health problems because of a history of excess acid-ash food intake being so common, then:

- Decrease your carbohydrate and protein intake by about one-third
- Increase your fruit, salad and vegetable intake by about one-third
- Consult with a holistic doctor, preferably one versed in nutritional and emotional evaluation

––––––

Over-Acid or Over-Alkaline?

Just as a log of wood burned in your fireplace leaves a mineral-ash, food ash refers to the minerals remaining after metabolizing foods in your tissues:

- Fruits and vegetables **alkalinize** tissues
- Proteins and carbohydrates **acidify** tissues

You are usually over-acid due to:

- Accumulated metabolic waste-acids
- Deficient fruit, salad and vegetable intake
- Excessive protein and carbohydrate intake

You need to estimate the ratio of foods you are eating: generally, eat the following *approximate* ratio of foods for your health:

50% *Alkaline-ash* foods (fruits, salads, vegetables)

50% *Acid-ash* foods (complex carbohydrates like starches, grains, cereals, breads, flour products; and proteins)

Approximate your food ratios. On any particular day it does not matter if one meal is mostly alkaline, and another is acid—just try to balance it out for the day! If you make a mistake, forget it and try again tomorrow. It is a subjective call that you make. It is what you do over weeks and months that makes the difference to your health—not on any few days.

The net result is that the Fat types require the plan presented in this chapter for health restoration.

[The following chart shows the fat types, their acid-alkaline reactions, and the percentage of raw foods needed for their healing.]

Fat Types

Acid/Alkaline Genetics Dietary-Ash and Raw Food Needs

———

This chart shows the Rocine types, their acid or alkaline food needs, and the percentage of raw foods needed for your health and healing.

BODY TYPE	ACID/ALKALINE GENETICS	% DIET ASH	% RAW FOODS
Barotic	*Intermediate*	*50:50*	*50*
Carboferic	*Intermediate*	*50:50*	*50*
Hydripheric	*Intermediate*	*50:50*	*30*
Isogenic	*Intermediate*	*50:50*	*30*
Lipopheric	*Intermediate*	*50:50*	*50*
Oxypheric	*Intermediate*	*50:50*	*50*
Pargenic	*Acid*	*70% alkaline*	*30*

Note that the above percentages will vary depending on aging and the health of individual types.

Notes

- Never eat foods you are allergic to, no matter what I recommend here; if you suspect allergy to a suggested food, eliminate it.
- Minimize your white sugar and alcohol intake.
- Eat the right foods most of the time and the diet will help you; you do not have to live out of a health food store (although such foods are healthier).
- All food lists are in descending order of concentration and value to you as a mineral source; whenever possible, choose foods in the upper half of each list first! One serving is ½ cup.
- If desired, you may interchange lunches for dinners.
- Avoid all junk foods, white sugar, foods with added sugar, and high fructose corn syrup

———

General Food Guide

Breakfasts

[Superimpose the nutritional information from your

EGGS (1-2) with lettuce, tomato, whole grain toast — 1-3 times/week; or

FRUIT SALAD, fresh with citrus fruit and a protein source (low-sugar yogurt, kefir, milk, cottage cheese, cheese, seeds or nuts) — 2-4 times/week; or

COOKED CEREALS, fruit, seeds, whole grain, and nuts — 2-5 times/week; or

OTHER —0-1 times/week

Eat unlimited fruit, salads, vegetables, with seeds/nuts for snacks. Wheat is a common allergy: avoid white and wheat breads; eat rye, sour dough, or oat breads instead

* * *

DAILY LIQUIDS

Pure water —as desired (except Hydripheric type)
Fruit and vegetable juices — 0-2 cups
Coffee, caffeine teas — 0-2 cups

[Include selections from your type mineral needs with each meal.]

Lunches

SALADS, mixed green, and 2-4 oz., of protein (fish, poultry, egg, cheese, tofu, seeds or nuts, etc.) [Dressings: use canola or olive oil* and vinegar; or low-fat/calorie dressing] — 2-4 times/week; or

VEGETABLES (steamed) with salad, and yogurt, or cottage cheese (or other breakfast proteins) — 1-2 times/week; or

FRUIT SALAD (see breakfast) — 0-1 times/week

SANDWICH, whole grains with a non-flesh protein (egg, tofu, cheese, etc.) —1-3 times/week; or

POULTRY, FISH, 3-4 oz., with a mixed green salad and/or steamed vegetables (or as a sandwich) —1-2 times/week; or

OTHER — 0-1 times/week

* Other oils less ideal; soybean is common allergen; minimize commercial dressings

[Include selections from your type mineral needs with each meal.]

Dinners

LEAN POULTRY OR FISH *(4-6 oz.)*
— *2-4 times/week*

PASTA, PROTEIN *(as above)*
—*1-3 times/week*

VEGETARIAN MEAL, *including legumes, tofu, cheese, cottage cheese, seeds or nuts, egg, etc.*
—*2-4 times/week*

LEAN BEEF *(4-6 oz.) — 0-2 times/month*

OTHER — *0-2 times/week*

Take all of the above with: mixed green salad, dressing (as before), and/or vegetables (steamed are best).

DESSERTS

Fruits, fresh — as desired
Low-sugar, healthy desserts — 0-3 times/week

If you have blood fat problems, cholesterol or triglycerides, eliminate all beef from your diet, and see my earlier books.

Eat fruit, unlimited salads and vegetables with seeds/nuts, low-sugar yogurt for snacks.

[Include selections from your type mineral needs with each meal.]

Fat Types Notes

Do not eat flesh everyday: have it on alternate days only. For munchies, have low calorie items like celery and other vegetables, along with yogurt and cottage cheese, etc. Some of you abuse your beef and red meat intake, perhaps several times weekly—this is a false craving; use your will to combat it if you want to be healthier!

Steamed Vegetables —Minerals are lost in the boiling of vegetables; best is steaming or wok cooking.

Minimize Foods — Only eat them 0-1 times/week! Be sure to eat the recommended foods to help your healing;

Food Combinations —Eating proteins at the same meal with starches often results in indigestion, gas or constipation (along with low blood sugar and making fat). Watch how this inharmonious food combination may be affecting you.

Minimize —
- All fatty foods
- Milk and dairy foods (unless otherwise noted)
- Commercial, sugared, and fatty salad dressings

- Beef, sugar, wines, alcohol, coffee, white sugar, red meats, and processed meats

Vegetarian Proteins — If you choose to be vegetarian, it will help your health after middle-age; because you have semi-carnivorous genes be sure to take a protein supplement of 20-30 grams/day (e.g., soy or egg-white powder in juice).

Healthy Weight — Invariably you hold excessive weight, and in addition to body type factors there may be a medical problem behind your fat storage. By eating according to your body type, you slowly and naturally lose excess weight! Accumulating evidence indicts high fructose corn syrup as a major cause of increased weight and obesity. Avoid it!

You have a sluggish fat-burning metabolism, and may have an under-active adrenal, thyroid, or pituitary gland resulting in hypoglycemia, and in this instance may need the services of a holistic doctor *(see Appendix* and my earlier books).

In Conclusion

I hope you have enjoyed reading this book. You should now know your body type and have learned some valuable information about how to be a healthier you! Do not forget the advice on page 10, along with my previous books on healing yourself.

If you desire further help or information with your body type or health from a holistic viewpoint, email me from page one of my web page:
Dr.Stenbeck.net

Good health and good luck!

———

Appendix

Brief Extracts from
The 22 Unique Body Types

Appendix A

Types
(Brief extract)

Type comes from 'typus' meaning an image or impression, the study of types being called typology.

▶ *Rocine: "A combination of mental and structural features is consistently found in people of the same type."*

Rocine wrote that all types are a mixture of positive and negative qualities. He based his work on the biochemical individuality of our *mineral* absorption and utilization. Of course, all minerals are absorbed, but he postulated that different types of people *selectively* absorb certain minerals, to a greater or lesser extent, requiring specific mineral foods for their enhanced health and healing.

▶ *The type information cannot predict what or who you will become, or how successful or not, but your type is capable of bringing a creative excellence to whatever you do in life. If your type has negative qualities that you disagree with, remember that they are only tendencies and may or may not manifest in you.*

This book enlarges on Rocine's premise (early 1900's), integrated with the later research of Herbert Sheldon, M.D., Ph.D., at Harvard University (1930's), along with my fifty years of observations and experience with this subject.

Comparing your shared physical (and sometimes psychological) descriptions with the Celebrity Lists further assists the identification of your type. It is not that you will look exactly like, or be a twin to, any particular celebrity. Look closely at a celebrity's features: face, profile, height, weight, head, etc. If you know something about their talents, beliefs, success and failure spheres, health and weight challenges, attitudes and behaviors, etc., then you get clues as to what your type may be.

———

Understanding Types and Sub-Types

Each of us has a clearly discernible dominant type. Visualize the celebrity examples from movies, politics, sports, the arts and public life, and try to identify with their physical features. Look for similar features, remembering that you will not recognize all attributes in yourself. You are not looking for your twin!

The sub-type issue is the main reason people of the same major type can look so different. Remember that a type description does not characterize you exactly, but depicts your individual variant of a type.

▶ *The type questionnaire pinpoints the major features of that type: if the celebrity examples are unhelpful, you may be an unusual variant (in which case ignore the celebrity issue and give yourself 7 points on Question 1).*

Minerals

Minerals are essential life nutrients that accelerate enzyme and chemical reactions and provide a basis for your body typing. Although found in all tissues, different minerals tend to be concentrated in certain organs, their presence or absence contributing to the healing of such tissues; e.g., zinc accelerates prostate healing; calcium and manganese promote bone, joint and connective tissue healing.

Specific foods nurture each type, some people needing meats for their health others needing a vegetarian diet. A high potassium diet nurtures one person, while another needs high sulfur, calcium, zinc, or another mineral.

Mineral Digestion and Absorption

Compared to vitamins, minerals are *difficult* to digest, absorb, and utilize. In people with strong digestive systems, this aspect may not be important. The following factors should be in place for optimal mineral metabolism:

1. Stomach Hydrochloric Acid Production
2. Parathyroid Hormone Balance
3. Organ Toxic Metal and Chemical Removal
   [See details in The 22 Unique Body Types.]

––––––

Total Body Healing

Note that from a holistic healing perspective, in addition to minerals and type information, the following healing factors are necessary:

> *Nutrient Balance*
> *Mental Balance*
> *Emotional Balance*
> *Spiritual Balance*
> *Detoxifying Integrity*

The above factors are all important to your total healing especially if you are interested in self-healing (see my earlier books).

––––––

Appendix B

Researchers
(Brief extract)

The predominant workers in this area of human individuality from around 1880's to the 1960's are Herbert Sheldon, M.D., Ph.D., Roger Williams, Ph.D., and Victor Rocine, D.Sc.

Much information on Sheldon's research exists on-line and in medical psychology libraries; for interested readers there are other lines of research published in the last century. This present book is primarily about Rocine's body types.

Herbert Sheldon M.D., Ph.D.

In contrast to Rocine, Sheldon at Harvard University in the 1930's was trained in the scientific method and did painstaking research and publishing on human individuality. In comparing his findings with Rocine's work, a direct putative correlation is visible.

Roger J. Williams, Ph.D.

Another significant researcher in human individuality is the renowned scientist and biochemist, Roger J. Williams. He demonstrated that different people have varying levels of nutrients, enzymes, and other metabolic chemicals in their bloodstreams.

▶ *Williams's research firmly expands on the premise of individual nutritional needs in human beings. If interested in his research, I highly recommend his book Biochemial Individuality.*

Victor Rocine, D.Sc.

Note that when a negative feature is indicated, say neurotic tendencies, all members of the type are <u>not</u> that way; it is a type tendency reported by Rocine.

Rocine studied type-related diseases finding links between mineral and dietary factors with individual types and their diseases. In each body type, one or more dominant minerals are preferentially absorbed and utilized over other minerals.

He recognized discrete body types from their physical appearance finding genetically based mineral dominance to be the determining feature. He also correlated their physical features with psychological characteristics.

———

Appendix C

Genetics, Types, and Diet
(Brief extract)

This section deals with how nervous system genetics helps determine your eating choices for health: you are either born to be a predominant meat eater, a partial or complete vegetarian, or something between the two. The genetic factor determining this dietary aspect is the *sympathetic and parasympathetic* components of your central nervous system. This represents a basic factor in eating for health.

This chapter helps you understand your dietary inheritance, although instinctively, you may already have arrived there!

- If born **sympathetic** dominant you are *genetically acid*, desiring a predominantly *vegetarian* diet for your health (about 70% fruit, salad, vegetables to 30% proteins and carbohydrates).

- If born **parasympathetic** dominant you are *genetically alkaline*, desiring a predominantly *carnivorous* diet for your health (about 70% proteins, carbohydrates to 30% fruits, salads, vegetables). Few of you ever choose to become vegetarian because of the difficulty in satisfying your protein needs without meats.

- If born ***intermediate*** dominant you may eat food groups with little concern for the acid/alkaline factor. However, after age 40, you need a semi-vegetarian diet for healthy eating.

———

Chart of Relative Nervous System Dominance

In the following Chart, if you relate to many of the symptoms on one side you probably have that nervous system dominance; relating to both sides indicates *Intermediate* dominance.

If Vegetarian (Over-acid) --
Eat 70% fruits, salads, vegetables
And 30% proteins, carbohydrates

If Carnivore (Over-alkaline) --
Eat 70% proteins, carbohydrates
And 30% fruits, salads, vegetables

If Intermediate --
Eat 50:50 of acid and alkaline-ash foods

Make an *approximate* estimate of your daily acid and alkaline food intake (such ratios varying from type to type).

———

Symptoms of Relative Genetic Dominance

Vegetarians (Over-acid)	**Carnivores** (Over-alkaline)
Sympathetic Dominance	Parasympathetic Dominance
little or no flesh desire	desire flesh
easily constipated	rarely constipated
slow digestion	fast digestion
easily dehydrated	not dehydrated
strong thirst	low thirst
pale face	flushed face
high pulse after food	slow pulse after food
easy gag reflex	slow gag reflex
cool dry skin	moist warm skin
nervous stomach	calm stomach
little eyelid blinking	much blinking
nervous tendency	mostly calm
slower healing	faster healing
low oxygen-uptake	good oxygen-uptake
easily breathless	seldom breathless
insomnia common	sleep easier
few muscle cramps	some night cramps
calcium deposits rare	get calcium deposits

Appendix D

Help Identifying your Body Type with Dr. Stenbeck

If you desire help in identifying your body type, follow these instructions, and answer the questionnaire. For further information and fees, send me an email from page one of the website:

DrStenbeck.net

First name: _____

Country of birth: _____

Upload photos and send to the above website:

- Head and shoulders: front and side views

- Full body: front and side views

- Also 1-2 teenage views

- If possible, casual photos of mother, father, siblings

MY TYPE CLASS MAY BE: _____

   (Thin, Muscle, or Fat)

AGE   -   _____

HEIGHT   -   _____ feet/inches

MY WEIGHT -   _____ pounds

   Heaviest at age: _____

- Lightest as adult: _____

- Estimate age 15: _____

VISION - Excellent Average   Poor:

HAIR - Natural color: _____

    - Thin/thick? _____

    - balding? _____

SKIN - Quality: _____

    - History of acne, boils, other:

_____

_____

TEETH   - Strong   Weak   Dentures

       - Cavity history: Many   Moderate   Few

MUSCLES - Strong   Average   Weak

    Sports played _____

JOINTS   - Strong   Average   Weak

HEALTH - Childhood diseases?

_____

_____

- Adult diseases?

_____

AVERAGE DIET

- Beef   _____ (times/week)

 - Poultry   _____ (times/week)

- Fish   _____ (times/week)

- Eggs   _____ (times/week)

- Water   _____ (glasses/day):

- Vegetarian? Vegan?   _____

- Other?   _____

- Did your childhood diet differ? _____

The above will help me know who you are! I will send you a follow-up questionnaire for further help in identifying your body type.

Appendix E

On-line Health Consultation with Dr. Stenbeck

For further information, or to comment on this book, or to receive a response on any health issue from a holistic viewpoint, send an email inquiry from page one of my website:

DrStenbeck.net

Following that, I will suggest further healing needs, which we may pursue with an on-line consult.

———

Appendix F

Notes

See my book <u>*The 22 Unique Body Types,*</u> available at the usual online source, for further information and details on all of the 22 Types. The Appendix in that book has further information about:

Mineral Functions and Food Sources

Further Reading

———